SPIRITUAL
HERBAL
HEALING

Beginning of herbalism

By

Lucy Steve

1st edition

ACKNOWLEDGEMENT

Praise be to God almighty for his mighty works and knowledge.

DEDICATION

This book is dedicated to God almighty for his gifts

Copyright ©

TABLE OF CONTENT

INTRODUTION

In this book we will be talking about some of the natural gift given to us by nature and their spiritual healings, Nature gifts these are natural resources blessed by GOD almighty on to us for all of our uses these gift come in different ways, forms, shape and method some of these gifs are known as spice,herb, charcoal, petroleum,trees etc these natural gift are not just use as food or medical use but can also use as spiritual awakening, cleanance soul lifting etc. In this book we will talk about some common plants that can be used in more than just one way.

These are plants that can be used in more than one way in our home.

Spiritual herbal healing is a holistic approach to wellness that combines the use of herbs and plants with spiritual or energy-based practices to promote physical, mental, and emotional well-being. It is rooted in the belief that there is a deep connection between the human spirit or soul and the natural world.

Key points about spiritual herbal healing:

1. **Herbal Remedies**: Herbal healing involves the use of specific plants, herbs, and botanicals for their therapeutic properties. These natural remedies are believed to have the power to address various physical and emotional ailments.

2. Spiritual Connection:

Practitioners of spiritual herbal healing often view these remedies as a means to not only address physical symptoms but also to align the individual with spiritual or energetic forces. This can include practices like prayer, meditation, or rituals.

3.Cultural and Traditional Roots:

Spiritual herbal healing is often deeply rooted in cultural and traditional practices. Different cultures have their unique approaches to using herbs and spirituality for healing.

4. **Holistic Approach:** It takes a holistic approach to health, considering the interconnectedness of mind, body, and spirit. It aims to bring balance and harmony to all aspects of an individual's well-being.

5.**ComplementaryPractice** Spiritual herbal healing is often used in conjunction with conventional medicine, as complementary or alternative therapies. It's essential for individuals to consult with trained practitioners and healthcare professionals to ensure safe and effective use.

6.**Personalized Healing** Practitioners often tailor treatments to the individual's specific needs and spiritual beliefs, making it a highly personalized approach to healing.

Overall, spiritual herbal healing is a practice that bridges the gap between the physical and spiritual realms, using the power of nature to promote health and well-being while acknowledging the significance of one's inner self and connection to the universe.

Types of plant

Grain of paradise (alligator pepper)

- Sweet bay   (bay leaves)
- Cinnamon
- Lemon grass
- Prekese
- Bitter kola
- Kolanut
- Tyme

Alligator pepper.

Thisi grain of paradise is also known as alligator pepper.Alligator Pepper is a West African edible spicy fruit in the form of small seeds covered in pods.

This plant is used as a spice in some countries but this plant has more uses than just cooking. Alligator pepper has a wide range of uses in food! In West Africa, it's commonly used as a spice for soups, stews, and sauces. It can also be used as a condiment or sprinkled on top of dishes. Alligator pepper has a pungent, peppery flavor that can add a nice kick to any dish. It's also used in traditional medicine to treat various ailments. In the eastern part of Nigeria, kola nuts are served alongside Alligator Pepper and alcohol to entertain visitors.

FACT ABOUT ALLIGATOR PEPPER

Botanical Name	Aframomum Melegueta
Other Names	Grains of Paradise, Mbongo spice, Hepper Pepper, Ossame, Melegueta, Pepper, Guinea

grains, Fom Wisa, or Guinea pepper.

Origin	West Africa
Pod Colour	Reddish-Brown
Pod Shape	Ovoid Fig-shaped capsules
Taste	Peppery-Warm

What Is The Local Name For Alligator Pepper In Nigeria?

Alligator Pepper is called Atare in the Yoruba language, ósè ójị́ in the Igbo language, and Chitta in the Hausa language. It is called alligator pepper because it has a seed bump that looks like that of an alligator back. Traditionalists say that the spiritual meaning of alligator pepper is water of the spirit as it is difficult to cook

without water.

USES OF ALLIGATOR PEPPER

Alligator pepper has a lot of Culinary and spiritual uses.

Some of the culinary uses of Alligator pepper includes using it as a spice to spice up foods like chicken, lamb, cake. And using it flavoring in alcoholic drinks like beer, ale and gin.

Also, alligator pepper is commonly used for spiritual jobs like protection from evil attacks, guns and poison. And also for the treatment of physical and spiritual diseases. It has spiritual awakening, cleanance of soul and used to renew charm.

Alligator pepper, also known as "Aframomum melegueta," is a spice commonly used in various regions, particularly in West Africa. It has several traditional and culinary uses:

1. CULINARY USES

SPICE: Alligator pepper is used as a spice to add a pungent and spicy flavor to a wide range of dishes, including soups, stews, and sauces.

SEASONING: It is often used to season meat, fish, and vegetables, enhancing the taste of dishes.

2. TRADITIONAL MEDICINE:

Digestive Aid: In some cultures, alligator pepper is believed to aid digestion and alleviate digestive issues.

It may be used to treat indigestion and bloating.

Antimicrobial Properties: It is thought to have antimicrobial properties and is sometimes used in traditional medicine for its potential to combat infections.

Aphrodisiac: Alligator pepper is sometimes considered an aphrodisiac and is used for its alleged ability to enhance sexual vitality.

3.RITUALS AND CEREMONIES:

Cultural Significance: Alligator pepper is used in various rituals and ceremonies in West African cultures. It is often included as part of traditional offerings and gifts during rituals, weddings, and other cultural events.

4.PRESERVATION AND FLAVORING:

Food Preservation: Alligator pepper is believed to have preservative properties and is used in some regions to help preserve certain types of food.

5. SCENT AND PERFUMERY:

Aromatic Uses: The seeds of alligator peqpper release a pleasant aroma when crushed or ground, making them sometimes used in perfumery and for their aromatic qualities.

It's important to note that the use of alligator pepper can vary widely from one culture to another, and its potential health benefits and properties are a subject of ongoing research. While it has cultural and culinary significance, individuals should be mindful of personal sensitivities or allergies when using this spice and consult with healthcare professionals for any medicinal applications.

HEALTH BENEFITS OF ALLIGATOR PEPPER

Here are some of the potential health benefits of using alligator pepper.

1. Weight Loss

Some research studies show that alligator pepper can help in fat loss and in boosting metabolism. For example, given a woman's daily dose of alligator pepper the woman will lose some fat and if the same is given to a man his metabolism will increase rapidly.

2. May Help Remedy Erectile Dysfunction

Alligator pepper has long been regarded as an aphrodisiac in traditional medicine.

A modern scientific study showed that alligator pepper may help inhibit enzymes that might contribute to erectile dysfunction

3. May Help Boost Testosterone

Some animal studies have shown Alligator pepper to help boost testosterone. Like a study done on rat given alligator pepper saw a significant increase in T levels

That said, more human trial is needed to ascertain alligator pepper's testosterone-boosting effect on humans.

4. Anti-Diabetes Property

West African Medicine has long used Alligator pepper for managing diabetes.

5. Anti-Poison Properties

Scientists suspect that Alligator pepper may contain anti-poison properties due to its antioxidant content, which can suppress inflammatory responses.

A study carried out on rats found out that rats that were given Alligator pepper were protected from a common research liver poison, carbon tetrachloride

6. Antibacterial Property

Compounds in Alligator pepper extract (like phenolic and diterpenes) has been scientifically shown to inhibit the growth of a wide range of bacteria like *Staphylococcus aureus, Listeria monocytogenes, Klebsiella pneumonia, Escherichia coli,* and so on.

6. Help Treat Skin Infections

Due to Alligator pepper's antibacterial action, it is widely used to treat various skin infections like chickenpox, measles and smallpox

7. Treatment Of Stomach & Intestinal Issues

Alligator pepper extract is potent in taking care of a range of gastrointestinal problems like bloating, constipation, ulcer, and stomach pain. It also aids food digestion.

8. Treatment Of Wound

The high quantity of tannin found in Alligator pepper makes it an excellent wound healer. It is effective in not just healing wounds but treating burns too.

9. Analgesic Properties

Alligator pepper extract is analgesic in nature which can be quite useful in relieving all sorts of pains including toothache, joint pain, rheumatoid pain and so on.

10. Aphrodisiac Properties

Studies have shown that alligator pepper is a potent aphrodisiac in both males and females.

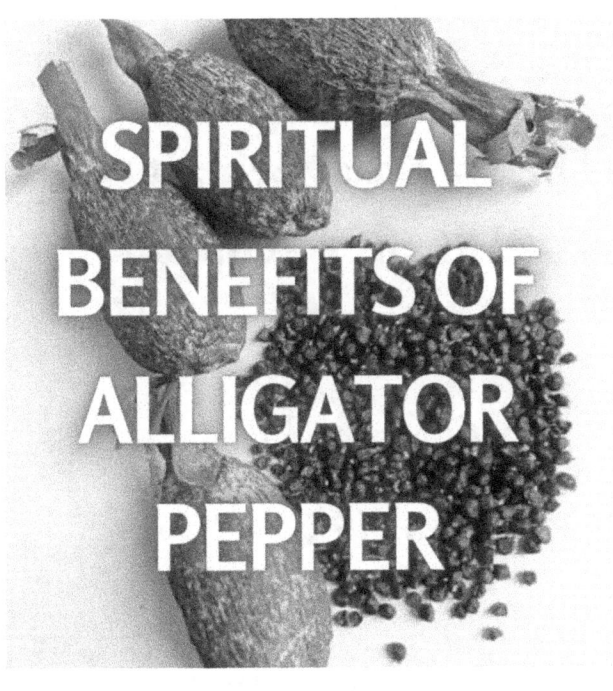

SPIRITUAL BENEFITS OF ALLIGATOR PEPPER

The Spiritual Benefits Of Alligator Pepper:

How To Use It To Obtain Amazing Results

The 10 spiritual benefits of alligator pepper are listed below.

1. Protection from evil spirits: Alligator pepper is believed

to provide spiritual protection from negative energy and evil spirits.

2. Good luck and prosperity: The seed is used in rituals to **bring good luck and prosperity** to individuals and families.

3. Enhancing spiritual awareness: Alligator pepper is believed to enhance spiritual

awareness and psychic abilities.

4. Connecting with ancestors: It is used in rituals and ceremonies to help connect with ancestors and the spiritual realm.

5. Warding off evil: It is believed that using alligator pepper can ward off evil spirits and **bad luck**.

6. Healing: Some people believe that alligator pepper has healing properties and can be used to treat a variety of ailments.

7. Strength and vitality: Alligator pepper is believed to give strength and vitality to those who consume it.

8. Purity: Some people believe that consuming

alligator pepper can purify the body and mind.

9. Love and fertility: It is also used as an aphrodisiac in some cultures, and is believed to increase love and fertility.

10. **Spiritual cleansing:** It is used as a spiritual cleanser and is believed to remove negative energy from the body.

More Benefits Of Alligator

Pepper

1. Alligator pepper is believed to have protective properties that guard against negative energy and vibrations. It is said to have the ability to both block and redirect any malevolent forces.

2. Alligator pepper has the potential to disrupt and neutralize charms when used alone, without the need for any additional ritual objects. Its mere presence is believed to be enough to bring about the desired outcome.

3. Alligator pepper has both destructive and protective properties. It has the potential to harm as well as **heal**. It can be used to take someone's life as well as to save one.

4. In reality, Alligator pepper plays a significant role in spiritual practices. It is considered unique among spiritual seeds for its perceived ability to purify individuals simply through consumption.

5. Eating and drinking in dreams can often lead to disappointment and a poor start to the day. Using Alligator pepper upon waking can help prevent this negative outcome.

6. As we journey through life, it's common to come across unwanted obstacles. Even on the brightest of paths, such as Broadway, we may experience setbacks in the form of cobwebs across our faces that can cause disappointment. However, it is believed that using Alligator pepper can aid in our recovery and help us move forward.

How to use alligator pepper spiritually

Warding off evil spirit : by putting seeds in every corner of your house

If don't feel comfortable for you upcoming journey put few seed of alligator pepper in your bag for protection.

1.If you have doubts about embarking on a trip, carry 7 seeds in your pocket. Upon returning, discard the seeds as a symbol of letting go of your uncertainty.

2. If you frequently experience terrible dreams or demonic attacks, place four of them at the four corners of your home.

3. If you believe your business is facing spiritual challenges, try this ritual: chew 7 or 4 seeds, but do not swallow them. As you chew, recite specific words or phrases. Repeat this process for 4 or 7 days, and you will likely notice a positive change in the energy of your business.

Please remember that the number of seeds and pills you take corresponds to the number of days they must be taken for. For example, if you take seven seeds, they must be taken for seven days, and if you take four pills, they must be taken for four days.

4. Regarding spiritual well-being, if you have a close relationship with someone you dislike or are not familiar with, use the numbers 4 or 7 to recite

powerful declarations while swinging them above your head. Then, set them aside.

5. If you come across strange feces in front of your residence, simply mix alligator pepper and **bitter kola** over it and then rinse it away. This will **send it back** to its sender.

6. To protect yourself from witches who may be stalking you, combine ground alligator pepper seeds with crushed ogirisi leaves. Mix this with original palm kernel oil and place the mixture on the door post of your home. It can be done anytime

7. If someone has deeply offended you and you are innocent, use alligator pepper and kola nuts, face the sun, and express your thoughts. Afterwards, dispose of the items. Your request has been acknowledged.

By incorporating Alligator pepper into your daily routine, you will start to see positive **changes in your life**. We would move to other natural resources that have spiritual benefits now.

Bay leaves

Bay leaf is an herb that is commonly used in cooking. It comes from the bay tree (Laurus nobilis), which is commonly found in the Mediterranean region. Bay leaf, also known as sweet bay or bay laurel, is an aromatic herb that's commonly used in cooking. The leaves are often dried and used to add flavor to soups, stews, and sauces. Bay leaves have a subtle, woody flavor that can add depth and complexity to dishes. They also have a long shelf life, so you can keep them on hand for a long time. Bay leaf is used by folk medicine chemicals in bay leaf might affect blood sugar and cholesterol level. Some people use Bay leaves for diabetic,common colds and many other conditions although it is not scientifically proven or supported. Did you know that bay leaves can also be used for things other than this?.

Use of bay leaf

Bay leaves, also known as "Laurus nobilis," are aromatic leaves commonly used in cooking for their distinctive flavor and aroma. Here are some common uses of bay leaves:

1. Culinary Uses:

Flavoring Soups and Stews: Bay leaves are often added to soups, stews, and sauces to infuse them with a subtle, earthy flavor.

Seasoning Meats: They are used to season various meats, such as beef, lamb, and poultry. Bay leaves can be added when roasting or braising.

Rice Dishes: Bay leaves are a key ingredient in dishes like rice pilaf and biryani, where they enhance the rice's fragrance and flavor.

Pickle Brine: Some people add bay leaves to pickle brine for extra flavor.

2. Aromatic Uses:

Aromatherapy: Bay leaves release a pleasant aroma when dried. They are sometimes used in potpourri, as natural air fresheners, or in aromatic sachets.

Herbal Teas: In some cultures, bay leaves are used to make herbal teas, often for their soothing and aromatic properties.

3. Medicinal and Health Benefits:

Digestive Aid: Bay leaves are believed to aid digestion and alleviate common digestive problems, such as indigestion and bloating. They are sometimes used in herbal remedies for these purposes.

4. Folklore and Superstitions:

Warding off Evil: In some cultures, bay leaves are believed to have protective qualities and are placed in households to ward off negative energies or evil spirits.

Good Luck:Bay leaves are considered symbols of good luck and are sometimes carried as talismans.

5. Insect Repellent:

- Bay leaves are believed to repel certain insects, such as moths and cockroaches. Placing bay leaves in pantries or kitchen cabinets is a traditional method of pest control.

It's important to note that while bay leaves are generally safe for culinary use and have a mild, pleasant flavor, they should not be consumed directly due to their tough and somewhat sharp texture. Bay leaves are typically removed from dishes before serving. Additionally, the health benefits attributed to bay leaves are often anecdotal, and their efficacy for medicinal purposes may vary from person to person.

SPIRITUAL USES OF BAY LEAF

1. Use bay leaves for protection & cleansing rituals

You may have tried smudging your space with Sage and even **Frankincense**, but did you know that you can burn a bay leaf for the same purposes? This sacred plant has been used for centuries in protective and aura-cleansing smudge rituals.

What's unique about the bay leaf is that it's flat and paper-thin; this means that you can write messages on the leaf before burning it, if you want to. If

you've been feeling worried, drained,
or negative lately, this ritual may work
perfectly for you! **Try writing your
worries in pen on a dried bay leaf,
and then burn it in a safe
container**. If you want, you can
include some sage or another sacred
plant or resin in there, as well.

As your bay leaves (and other desired
herbs) burn, imagine those stressors
floating away as the smoke dissipates.

You'll have a clear visual for the Universe absorbing your worries, and in addition, the bay leaf smoke will help to extract any negative energy from your space and your body.

2. Place a bay leaf in your wallet to attract wealth

Not only can you write your worries and stressors onto a bay leaf– you can also write down what you do want! **If**

you're hoping to attract wealth, try this ritual:

First, write your desires onto the bay leaf. Remember that these don't all have to revolve around money; "abundance" can also mean material objects, a healthy body, supportive community, and so on.

After writing down your desires, hold the bay leaf and visualize those desires.

Vividly imagine how you'll feel when you receive them. Take your time doing this.

When you're done, simply place the bay leaf in your wallet. Now, you'll carry around that energy of abundance everywhere you go! This will signal to the Universe that you're ready to receive all which you hope for.

3. Use a bay leaf for manifestation rituals

You can also try the above abundance ritual without tucking the bay leaf away in your wallet. Simply write your desires– what you'd like to manifest– on the bay leaf, as per the above point. Take plenty of time to visualize what you're manifesting with the bay leaf in your hand.

This time, instead of keeping the bay leaf, you'll burn it. Again, feel free to burn sage or anything else with your bay leaf. As your leaves burn, visualize your desires drifting upwards and becoming one with Source energy; then, allow Source to take care of your desires for you.

4. Drink bay leaf teas for stress relief & relaxation

Bay leaves might taste great in stews and soups, but you can prepare them as a tea, as well. The tea will taste slightly spicy, but if you're a fan of its aroma, it makes a powerful stress-relief and health-boosting tonic for everyday use.

Many bay leaf tea lovers swear by its calming effects. If you're anxiety-prone, try this tea once or twice a day and you may find that it gently soothes your frayed nerves and worried mind. This works for everyday use as well as for spiritual rituals. You may try a cup of bay leaf tea before meditation or yoga, or during a new or full moon ritual.

5. Place a bay leaf under your pillow for lucid dreams, clairvoyance, and astral travel

Bay leaves are widely known for their power to develop psychic abilities, and most commonly, what's known as the "clairs": clairvoyance, clairaudience, clairsentience, claircognizance, clairgustance and clairalience. In short, what this means is that bay leaves can help to heighten your extrasensory abilities, in order to receive psychic messages, communicate with your spiritual team, and connect to the Universe. You can sleep with a bay leaf under your pillow to receive psychic messages in your dreams.

This same method also helps with lucid dreaming or astral travel, both of which are difficult techniques but, once mastered, can help to connect you with ancestors.

6. Healing recipes: use bay leaf in soups and stews

If you browse recipes online, you'll notice that plenty of soups and stews call for a couple of bay leaves, as they add flavor and aroma to meals. You can, however, also cook with bay leaves to boost your overall health. Bay leaves contain loads of antioxidants, and they carry antimicrobial and anti-inflammatory properties, as well. So, next time you come down with a cold, trying a stew that contains bay leaves might help!

7. Use bay leaf during full and new moon rituals

Whether or not you already practice

any rituals around the moon cycle, bay

leaves are a great addition to your routines. We've talked above about using bay leaves to banish negative energy and to call in abundance these practices attract the best results when completed at the correct time of the moon cycle.

First of all, the new moon works best for manifestation, i.e. attracting abundance. When the new moon rolls around each month, use these rituals as described above: placing a bay leaf in your wallet, or burning a bay leaf with your desires written on it.

On the other hand, the full moon carries a strong energy for releasing all that is not serving you. Around the time of the full moon each month, try using the releasing rituals: use bay leaves to release negativity as described above, burn bay leaves to cleanse your space, or drink bay leaf tea to soothe

worry

8. Use salt & bay leaf for cleansing your body & space

Similar to clear quartz, **salt can work as an energetic cleanser** and as an amplifier of other spiritual tools (such as bay leaves). Thus, adding salt to any bay leaf ritual can make the practice even more powerful.

You might try placing bowls of sea salt dotted with bay leaves in every room of your home. In addition, you could take a bay leaf bath: add a cup of Sea Salt or Epsom Salt to your bath water, and throw in a few bay leaves. The salt and leaves will work together to create an energetically cleansing and **recharging bath,** and you'll get a delicious-smelling, spiritual spa-like experience.

9. Burn dried bay leaves to attract love

We've already discussed the magic of using bay leaves to manifest abundance, but "abundance" can also include love! If you're looking for an effortless, supportive romantic relationship, burning bay leaves can send a message to the Universe to attract that energy towards you.

The easiest way to do this is to simply write the word "love" on a bay leaf, and mindfully burn it, visualizing that intention of receiving love drifting up towards Source.

You can, however, get a little more detailed with your request. Affirmations work well in this case; ask yourself what exactly you're looking for in your desired relationship. Do you hope for emotional support? Adventure? Stability? Turn your wishes into an affirmation! This might sound something like: *"I love supporting and feeling supported by my loving partner!"*.

Write your affirmation on the bay leaf, and then follow the burning ritual: safely light your leaf, place it in a fire-safe container while it burns, and visualize the Universe receiving your request as the smoke drifts upwards.

It's important to remember that, when practicing love manifestation spells such as this one, it's not a good idea to write a person's name on the leaf in hopes of making that person love you back. The Universe can't make anyone love you – they have to choose it for themselves! Plus, it's healthy to remember this: you deserve a relationship that you don't have to beg for.

Growing bay leaf tree in your compand bring about good luck and positive energy to the environment and help balance the emotion of everything and everyone in the environment.

Cinnamon

Cinnamon is a spice that is made from the inner bark of trees scientifically known as *Cinnamomum*. Cinnamon is a spice that has been prized for its medicinal properties for thousands of years.

In recent years, modern science has started to confirm many of the potential health benefits associated with cinnamon.

Contains powerful medicinal properties

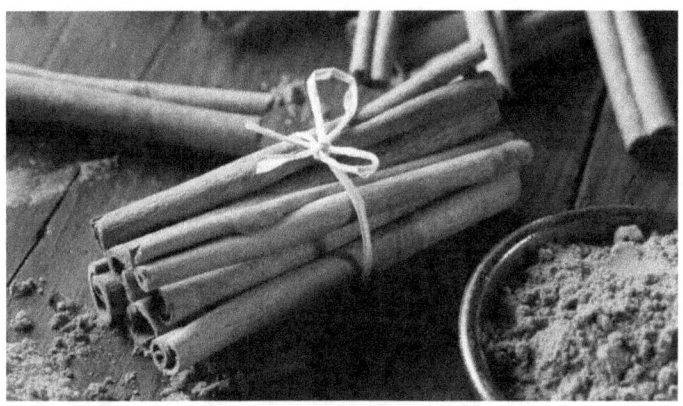

Cinnamon is a spice that is made from the inner bark of trees scientifically known as *Cinnamomum*.

It has been used as an ingredient throughout history, dating back as far as Ancient Egypt. It used to be rare and valuable and was regarded as a gift fit for kings

These days, cinnamon is affordable and widely available in most supermarkets. It's also found as an ingredient in various foods and recipes.

There are two main types of cinnamon

- **Ceylon cinnamon:** This type is also known as "true" cinnamon.

- **Cassia cinnamon:** This is the most common variety today and what people generally refer to as "cinnamon."

Cinnamon is made by cutting the stems of cinnamon trees. The inner bark is then extracted and the woody parts removed.

When it dries, it forms strips that curl into rolls, called cinnamon sticks. These sticks can be ground to form cinnamon powder.

The distinct smell and flavor of cinnamon are due to the oily part, which is very high in the compound cinnamaldehyde. Scientists believe that this compound is responsible for most of cinnamon's powerful effects on health and **metabolism**

2. Loaded with antioxidants

Antioxidants protect your body from oxidative damage caused by free radicals

Cinnamon is loaded with powerful antioxidants, including polyphenols

One study found that cinnamon supplementation could significantly increase antioxidant levels in the blood while reducing levels of markers used

to measure inflammation, such as C-reactive protein

In fact, the antioxidant effects of cinnamon are so powerful that it can

even be used as a natural food
preservative

3. May have anti-inflammatory
properties

Inflammation is incredibly important, as
it helps your body respond to infections
and repair tissue damage.

However, inflammation can become a problem when it's chronic and directed against your body's own tissues

Cinnamon may be useful in this regard. Studies show that this spice and its antioxidants have potent **anti-inflammatory** properties

- Special Diets

- Healthy Eating

- Food Freedom

- Conditions

- Feel Good Food

- Products

- Vitamins & Supplements

- Sustainability

- Weight Management

10 Evidence-Based Health Benefits of Cinnamon

Cinnamon is rich in antioxidants and other beneficial compounds. Some research suggests that it may help support blood sugar control, protect against heart disease, and reduce inflammation.

Cinnamon is a spice that has been prized for its medicinal properties for thousands of years.

In recent years, modern science has started to confirm many of the potential health benefits associated with cinnamon.

Cinnamon has several potential health benefits, although it's important to note that these effects may vary from person to person. Some of the potential benefits of cinnamon include:

rich in antioxidants, which can help protect your cells from oxidative damage caused by free radicals.

1.Antioxidant Properties: Cinnamon is rich in antioxidants, which can help protect your cells from oxidative damage caused by free radicals.

2. **Anti-Inflammatory:** It may have anti-inflammatory properties that can help reduce inflammation in the body.

3. **Blood Sugar Control:** Cinnamon may help improve insulin sensitivity, which can be beneficial for people with diabetes or those at risk of developing it. It may also help lower blood sugar levels.

4.Heart Health: Some studies suggest that cinnamon can improve various risk factors for heart disease, such as reducing bad LDL cholesterol and triglycerides.

5.Anti-Microbial: Cinnamon has natural antimicrobial properties that can help fight infections and inhibit the growth of bacteria and fungi.

6.Neurological Benefits: There is ongoing research into the potential cognitive and neuroprotective benefits of cinnamon, including its role in Alzheimer's disease prevention.

7. Weight Management: Cinnamon may help control appetite and contribute to weight loss efforts by stabilizing blood sugar levels.

8. Digestive Health: It can aid digestion and reduce discomfort from indigestion, bloating, and gas.

9.Anti-Cancer: Some studies suggest that cinnamon extracts may inhibit the growth of cancer cells, but more research is needed.

Remember that while cinnamon can be a healthy addition to your diet, it's essential to consume it in moderation. Excessive amounts can lead to health issues, and it's crucial to consult with a healthcare professional if you have specific health concerns or are considering using cinnamon supplements for therapeutic purposes.

Here are 10 health benefits of cinnamon that are supported by scientific research.

1. Contains powerful medicinal eproperties

Cinnamon is a spice that is made from the inner bark of trees scientifically known as *Cinnamomum*.

It has been used as an ingredient throughout history, dating back as far as Ancient Egypt. It used to be rare and valuable and was regarded as a gift fit for kings

These days, cinnamon is affordable and widely available in most supermarkets. It's also found as an ingredient in various foods and recipes.

There are two main types of cinnamon

- **Ceylon cinnamon:** This type is also known as "true" cinnamon.

- **Cassia cinnamon:** This is the most common variety today and what people generally refer to as "cinnamon." Cinnamon is made by cutting the stems of cinnamon trees. The inner bark is then extracted and the woody parts removed.

When it dries, it forms strips that curl into rolls, called cinnamon sticks. These sticks can be ground to form cinnamon powder. The distinct smell and flavor of cinnamon are due to the oily part, which is very high in the compound cinnamaldehyde.

Scientists believe that this compound is responsible for most of cinnamon's powerful effects on health and metabolism

Cinnamon is a popular spice. It's high in cinnamaldehyde, which is thought to be responsible for most of cinnamon's health benefits.

2. Loaded with antioxidants

Antioxidants protect your body from oxidative damage caused by free radicals Cinnamon is loaded with powerful antioxidants, including polyphenols

One study found that cinnamon supplementation could significantly increase antioxidant levels in the blood while reducing levels of markers used to measure inflammation, such as C-reactive protein

In fact, the antioxidant effects of cinnamon are so powerful that it can even be used as a natural food preservative

Cinnamon contains large amounts of highly potent polyphenol antioxidants.

3. May have anti-inflammatory properties Inflammation is incredibly important, as it helps your body respond to infections and repair tissue damage.

However, inflammation can become a problem when it's chronic and directed against your body's own tissues

Cinnamon may be useful in this regard. Studies show that this spice and its antioxidants have potent anti-inflammatory properties

The antioxidants in cinnamon have anti-inflammatory effects, which may help lower your risk of disease.

4. Could protect against heart disease.

Cinnamon has been linked to a reduced risk of heart disease, which is the leading cause of death around the globe

According to one review, supplementing with at least 1.5 grams (g), or about 3/4 of a teaspoon (tsp.), of cinnamon per day was able to reduce levels of triglycerides, total cholesterol, LDL (bad) cholesterol, and blood sugar in people with metabolic disease

Another review of 13 studies found that cinnamon could reduce triglyceride and total cholesterol levels, both of which are risk factors for heart disease

Cinnamon has also been shown to reduce blood pressure when consumed consistently for at least 8 weeks.

When combined, all of these factors could help reduce your risk of heart disease.

5. Could improve sensitivity to insulin

Insulin is one of the key hormones that regulate metabolism and energy use

It's also essential for transporting blood sugar from your bloodstream to your cells

However, some people are resistant to the effects of insulin. This is known as insulin resistance, a hallmark of conditions like metabolic syndrome and type 2 diabetes

While more research is needed, some studies suggest that cinnamon may be able to reduce insulin resistance

By increasing insulin sensitivity, cinnamon can lower blood sugar levels and support better blood sugar control

6. May have beneficial effects on neurodegenerative diseases

Neurodegenerative diseases are characterized by progressive loss of the structure or function of nerve cells

Alzheimer's and Parkinson's disease are two of the most common types

Certain compounds found in cinnamon appear to inhibit the buildup of a protein called tau in the brain, which is one of the hallmarks of Alzheimer's disease

In a 2014 study in mice with Parkinson's disease, cinnamon helped protect neurons, normalized neurotransmitter levels, and improved motor function

However, these effects need to be studied further in humans.

7. May prevent bacterial and fungal infections

Cinnamaldehyde, one of the main active components of cinnamon, may be beneficial against various kinds of infection.

Test-tube studies suggest that cinnamon oil could help kill certain fungi that cause respiratory tract infections

It may also inhibit the growth of certain bacteria, including *Listeria* and *Salmonella*

Plus, the antimicrobial effects of cinnamon may also help prevent tooth decay and reduce bad breath

However, the evidence is mostly limited to test-tube studies, so more research in humans is needed.

8.May have antiviral properties

Some research suggests that cinnamon may help protect against certain viruses.

For example, cinnamon extracted from Cassia varieties is thought to be beneficial against HIV-1, the most common strain of HIV in humans

Other studies suggest that cinnamon could also protect against other viruses, including influenza and

Dengue, a viral infection transmitted by mosquitoes

Still, additional human trials are needed to confirm these effects.

What Does Cinnamon Symbolize?

Native to Sri Lanka and Myanmar, cinnamon is a very positive herb that has been a **symbol of fertility, love, spirituality, protection, good luck and health for centuries**. Cinnamon represents masculine energy and is associated with the Sun and the element of Fire.

Cinnamon use was first recorded in Chinese writings dating back to 2800

BC. In China, cinnamon is associated with yang energy and is believed to have the power to increase the free flow of Chi (Qi) throughout the body that aid health and healing. In medieval times, cinnamon was famed for its healing properties and was used to heal a variety of ailments.

its ability to purify a space. Simply light your incense and walk around your room, allowing the smoke to enter every corner to dispel any negativity that has entered your home.

This process is also thought to promote physical healing, love, and success, as well as increasing your spiritual awareness which will help you to trust your own intuition. Throughout history, cinnamon has also been highly regarded as a herb that can raise spiritual awareness due to its high vibration. **Cinnamon has the power to activate the third eye chakra promoting physic awareness and intuition**.

Then just blow the cinnamon and salt from your hand into the room.

You can also burn cinnamon incense or candles anointed with cinnamon oil to encourage prosperity to enter your life. In addition, cinnamon is an excellent ingredient for any love spell as this herb is said to promote the release of Oxytocin (also known as the cuddle hormone).

1. Carry cinnamon with you for attracting good luck & wealth.

The high vibration of cinnamon makes it an excellent good luck charm that will also work to shield you from negative energies and spiritual attacks. **Carrying a stick of cinnamon in your wallet or purse, or even adding a few drops of cinnamon oil to the outside of your purse, is said**

to attract prosperity both on a physical level and on a spiritual level.

Other herbs that work well with cinnamon and increase its wealth attracting abilities are cloves, cardamom and nutmeg. So you can consider carrying a combination of these herbs (like one stick of cinnamon and a couple of cloves) to increase the power of cinnamon.

2. Use cinnamon + clove spray for protection

Just the thought of cinnamon is known to invoke a sense of warmth and homeliness. Making a simple cinnamon spray will allow you to invoke these feelings of protection whenever you feel lethargic, down, or when you feel like everything is going wrong in your life.

Simply put a handful of crushed cinnamon sticks and cloves into 300ml of boiled water and allow to infuse for a few minutes. Then spray the concoction (after pouring it in a spray bottle) in each of the four corners of your home and by the front door to increase prosperity and health, and to ward off negative energies. The magical properties of clove will work with the spiritual healing properties of cinnamon to shield your home in a protective and uplifting scent.

3. Burn cinnamon for cleansing and to dispel negative energy.

Cinnamon can be burned by placing powdered cinnamon or stick incense on a charcoal disc. You can also directly burn a cinnamon stick however do be careful to ensure you have a bowl for the burning embers to drop into.

Traditionally, cinnamon is almost as popular as white sage or **Palo Santo** in its ability to purify a space. Simply light your incense and walk around your room, allowing the smoke to enter every corner to dispel any negativity that has entered your home. This process is also thought to promote physical healing, love, and success, as well as increasing your spiritual awareness which will help you to trust your own intuition.

Alternatively you can put a couple of cinnamon sticks into boiling water and let the resulting steam circulate in different areas of your home that need cleansing. **You can also wash the floors of your home with cinnamon infused water.**

4. Place cinnamon sticks around your home for protection & to block negative energy.

If you are looking to create an effective protective barrier around your home, try tying cinnamon sticks together on a piece of string and hanging them above your front door. The most common number of sticks used is **nine** as it is a number that has spiritual significance in numerous cultures, including Buddhism and the Baha'i faith, and is believed to symbolize perfection, love, enlightenment, and compassion.

Aside from your front door, you can also place cinnamon sticks on your window sills if you are worried about negative energies entering through other areas of your home.

Alternatively, you can also sprinkle a few pinches of powdered cinnamon around your room and window sills for protection.

5. Diffuse cinnamon essential oil for raising your spiritual vibration

The high spiritual vibration of cinnamon can be used to increase your own vibrations and allow you to achieve a higher level of consciousness and understanding. This makes it an excellent herb to use during any meditation practice. **Raising your vibration** will also help you to feel more positive, fulfilled, and strong enough to tackle any situation that is thrown your way.

Its attractive aroma will encourage you to view situations in a positive and joyful light, which makes it a very beneficial herb if you suffer from depression, anxiety, or feelings of pessimism.

Simply add a few drops to a diffuser and take deep breaths to allow the intense scent to calm your mind and promote a sense of self-awareness and confidence. You can also mix 2-3 drops of cinnamon oil into your usual moisturizer and use it for a rejuvenating massage or simply to moisturize and invigorate your skin.

You can also add a few drops of cinnamon oil (or water infused with cinnamon) to your bath water which will help raise your vibration, increase passion, aid clarity and invite success into your life.

6. Drink cinnamon tea for healing, raising awareness & intuition

Cinnamon tea is usually prepared by boiling a small (around an inch) cinnamon stick in water and allowing it a few minutes to infuse the drink with its sweet scent.

Drinking a cup of cinnamon tea before any form of divination is thought to increase your spiritual awareness and allow for a more accurate reading. **It is an excellent beverage to drink when you first wake up in the morning to boost your mood and shift your consciousness into a more relaxed, confident, and receptive state ready for the day ahead!**

7. Use cinnamon blowing ritual for manifesting your desires

Cinnamon is a common ingredient added to any kind of spell work as it is believed to enhance your intent. **One of the simplest rituals for bringing prosperity and success into your life is through cinnamon blowing.**

Here's how to do the cinnamon blowing ritual:

Simply take a pinch of sea salt and a small amount of cinnamon powder in your dominant hand and take it to the place you wish to infuse with positive vibes, healing, or success, such as a workplace or your home. It is a good idea to close your eyes at this stage and focus on what you want to manifest; whether it be financial stability, physical healing, or simply to bless the space with good luck.

You can also say a few words aloud to solidify your intentions. For instance, ***"When this cinnamon blows, prosperity and good luck in this house will come in!"***

Then just blow the cinnamon and salt from your hand into the room.

You can also burn cinnamon incense or candles anointed with cinnamon oil to encourage prosperity to enter your life. In addition, cinnamon is an excellent ingredient for any love spell as this herb is said to promote the release of Oxytocin (also known as the cuddle hormone).

8. Use cinnamon during moon rituals to attract success and wealth

The light of a full moon is known to add power to any spell or ritual. **The tree from which cinnamon is harvested is believed to be ruled by the moon so it is a fantastic herb to use during any moon ritual.**

As cinnamon is a positive herb, it is best used in moon magic spells that focus on bringing success, wealth, and joy to your life but it is also very effective when used during protection spells. Central to cinnamon's magical properties is its connection to prosperity so it is particularly powerful during new moon rituals to signify your intentions for the month to come, and also for any spell that works to bring abundance into your life.

9. Use cinnamon to improve relationship with your significant other

To improve the relationship between you and your significant other, burn powdered cinnamon along with a pinch of powered sandalwood and myrrh and show the smoke around the rooms where you spend the maximum time together with your beloved. To enhance the effect, use an intention and recite a prayer as you show the smoke around.

You can also use cinnamon as an ingredient in love and protection spell jars to increase the effect of the spell/ritual.

10. Use cinnamon to increase your psychic and intuitive abilities

Burning cinnamon powder with **sandalwood powder** opens and activates your third eye chakra increasing your psychic abilities, focus and intuition. Do this before a meditative or divination session to attract new insights that will help change your life.

You can also dilute cinnamon essential oil (with a carrier oil) and use it to anoint your third eye chakra. Doing this every morning or night before going to bed can aid spiritual awareness and clarity.

Spiritual benefits of cinnamon

Cinnamon has been associated with various spiritual and cultural beliefs in different parts of the world. While its spiritual benefits are largely subjective and rooted in traditions, here are some common spiritual associations with cinnamon:

1. Purification and Cleansing: Cinnamon is believed to have purifying properties. In many spiritual and religious practices, it is used to cleanse spaces, objects, and even the human body. The aroma of cinnamon is thought to clear negative energy and invite positivity.

2. Protection: Cinnamon is often considered a protective herb. It is used to create a protective barrier or shield against negative influences, energies, or entities. Some people carry or wear cinnamon as an amulet for protection.

3.SpiritualAwareness: Cinnamon is said to enhance spiritual awareness and consciousness. It is believed to help individuals connect with their inner selves and higher spiritual realms during meditation and prayer.

4.Sensuality and Love: In some traditions, cinnamon is associated with sensuality and love. It is used to kindle passion and romance. Cinnamon may be included in love spells or rituals designed to attract romantic relationships.

5. Luck and Prosperity: Cinnamon is sometimes considered a symbol of good luck and prosperity. It is used in rituals and offerings to invoke positive energy and good fortune.

6.Enhancing Psychic Abilities: Some individuals believe that cinnamon can enhance psychic abilities, intuition, and clairvoyance. It is used to stimulate the third eye chakra and heighten spiritual insights.

It's important to note that the spiritual benefits of cinnamon are largely based on cultural and individual beliefs and may vary widely. These beliefs are not scientifically proven but are deeply rooted in tradition and spirituality. If you are interested in using cinnamon for spiritual purposes, it's essential to do so respectfully and in accordance with your own beliefs or the traditions of your culture or religion.

How to use cinnamon

spiritually

The use of cinnamon for spiritual or cultural purposes can vary widely, and the methods can be specific to individual beliefs or traditions. Here are some common ways to use cinnamon for spiritual purposes:

1. Cinnamon Incense:

Burn cinnamon sticks or powdered cinnamon as incense. The rising smoke is believed to carry the aromatic and purifying properties into the environment.

2. Candle Magic:

Carve symbols, words, or intentions into a candle, and then roll the candle in powdered cinnamon. As the candle burns, it is thought to release the energy and intentions associated with cinnamon.

3. Sprinkling or Dusting:

Sprinkle powdered cinnamon around your home, on thresholds, or in specific areas you wish to purify or protect. Some people use it to mark sacred spaces or altars.

4. Amulets and Talismans:

Carry a cinnamon stick or powder in a small pouch, or wear it as an amulet for protection, love, or good luck.

5. Meditation and Prayer:

Light a cinnamon-scented candle or incense while meditating or engaging in spiritual practices. Some individuals find that the aroma enhances their connection to higher spiritual realms.

6. Baths and Body Products: Add a

few drops of cinnamon essential oil or a cinnamon-infused bath salt to your bathwater to cleanse and purify your body and spirit.

7. Offerings:

In various spiritual and religious practices, cinnamon may be offered as a symbol of respect and gratitude to deities or spiritual entities.

8. Intentions and Affirmations:

As you use cinnamon in rituals, meditations, or prayers, set clear intentions or affirmations related to your spiritual goals or desires.

9. Cleansing Rituals:

Burn cinnamon incense or sprinkle powdered cinnamon in your home to cleanse the space of negative energies and invite positivity.

10. Protection Charms:

Create protective charms or amulets by carrying a cinnamon stick or pouch of powdered cinnamon with you for defense against negative influences.

11. Altar Decorations:Place cinnamon sticks or powder on your

spiritual altar as offerings to deities or as symbols of blessings and protection.

12. Meditation Enhancer:

Light a cinnamon-scented candle or incense during meditation to help enhance your focus and spiritual awareness.

13. Anointing Oil:

Mix cinnamon essential oil with a carrier oil to create anointing oil for rituals and blessings. Use it to anoint yourself or sacred objects.

14. Love Spells or Rituals:

Use cinnamon in rituals designed to attract love or deepen romantic connections. This might involve adding it to love potions or spells.

15. Prosperity and Luck:

Incorporate cinnamon into rituals or offerings aimed at attracting luck and prosperity into your life.

16. Dream Work:

Place a cinnamon stick or a sachet of cinnamon under your pillow to enhance dream recall and encourage spiritual insights.

17. Chakra Alignment: Use cinnamon to stimulate the third eye chakra, which is associated with intuition and spiritual awareness.

18. Intent-Infused Baths:

Add cinnamon-infused bath salts to your bathwater while setting intentions for spiritual growth, purification, or protection.

Remember that the way you use cinnamon spiritually should align with your own beliefs and intentions. It's essential to approach these practices with respect, mindfulness, and a clear sense of purpose. Additionally, consider any safety precautions or sensitivities to cinnamon when incorporating it into your spiritual rituals.

When using cinnamon for spiritual purposes, it's essential to do so with respect and mindfulness of your intentions and beliefs. The specific practices and rituals may vary, and you should follow what aligns with your personal spiritual or cultural traditions. Additionally, ensure safety when using cinnamon in any form, and be cautious if you have allergies or sensitivities to this spice.

CONCLUSION

Nature touch covers more pages. In the next volume we will talk more on the common spice and their spiritual benefits. If you enjoy this **edition** please comment for the next **edition** .

In conclusion, spiritual herbal healing is a holistic and culturally rooted approach that combines the therapeutic power of herbs with spirituality, aiming to promote overall well-being by addressing the physical, mental, and spiritual aspects of an individual's health. This practice underscores the deep connection between nature and the human spirit, offering a personalized and complementary pathway to healing and balance.

Thank you for reading. Reading is food for thought and soul the more you read the more you learn and ready to give out more knowledge or food for the soul.

www.ingramcontent.com/pod-product-compliance
Lightning Source LLC
Chambersburg PA
CBHW072202290526
45794CB00004B/1611